Dear Maxine,

May you always be happy.
May you always be healthy.
May you always feel like you belong.

Colleen Guanuale

Thanks to Chris, my husband for his encouragement!

Thanks to Erin, Deneen, Robin, and Mary for sharing my stories.

Thanks to Angela for editing.

Dedicated to my mother, Dorothy Etta McKnight Kamis, who always said to follow your passion.

Thanks to my grandchildren who are the characters in my books. (Jayde, Dylan, and Kylie)

Thanks to my children Michael and Kathleen for their support.

"The Magic Word"
Colleen Guanciale
Early Childhood

Kylie, Jayde, and Dylan have been inside all morning playing computer games. They decide it is time for something different, and Kylie suggests one of her favorite games, The Magic Word.

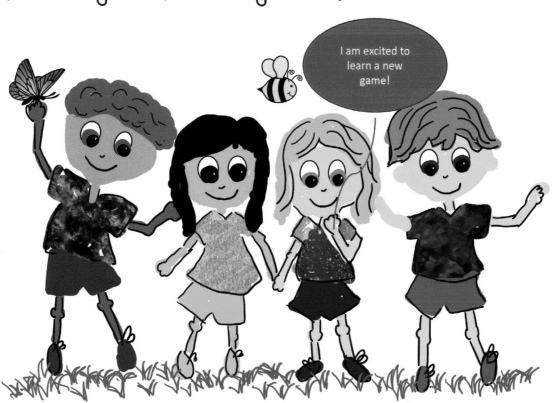

Kylie knows that to play a fair game,
she needs to explain the rules.
The rules are easy.

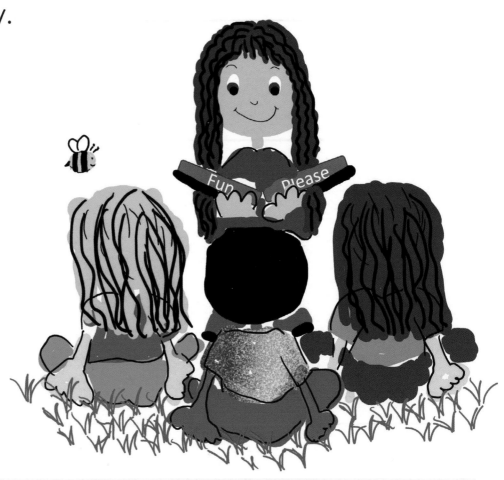

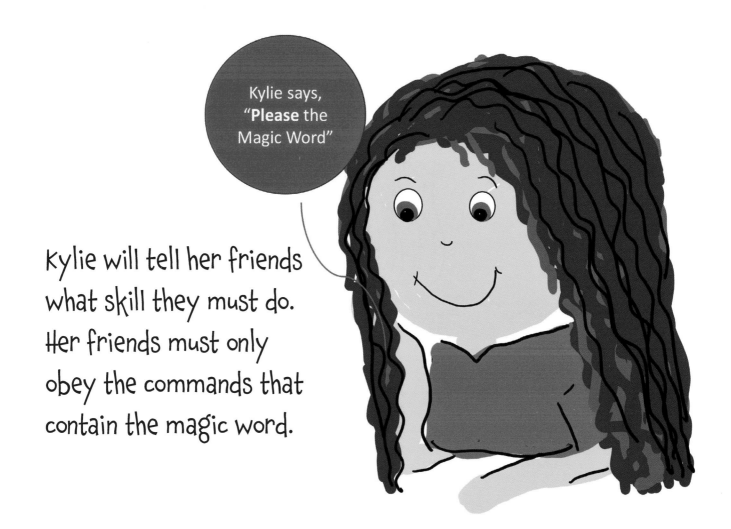

Kylie says, "**Please** the Magic Word"

Kylie will tell her friends what skill they must do. Her friends must only obey the commands that contain the magic word.

What do you think the magic word might be?

Could it be abracadabra?   Or shazam?

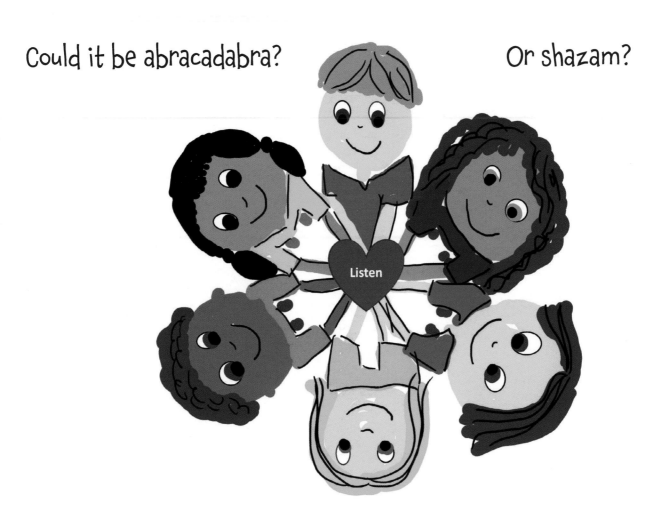

Kylie knows what it is – it is the word please!

Kylie would love for you to play along with her and her friends. She thinks you will have fun!

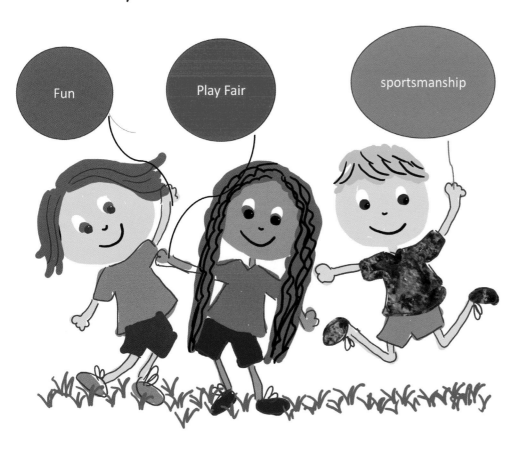

You will have to listen very carefully though because she will try her best to trick you. Make sure you only do the action when Kylie says, "Please."

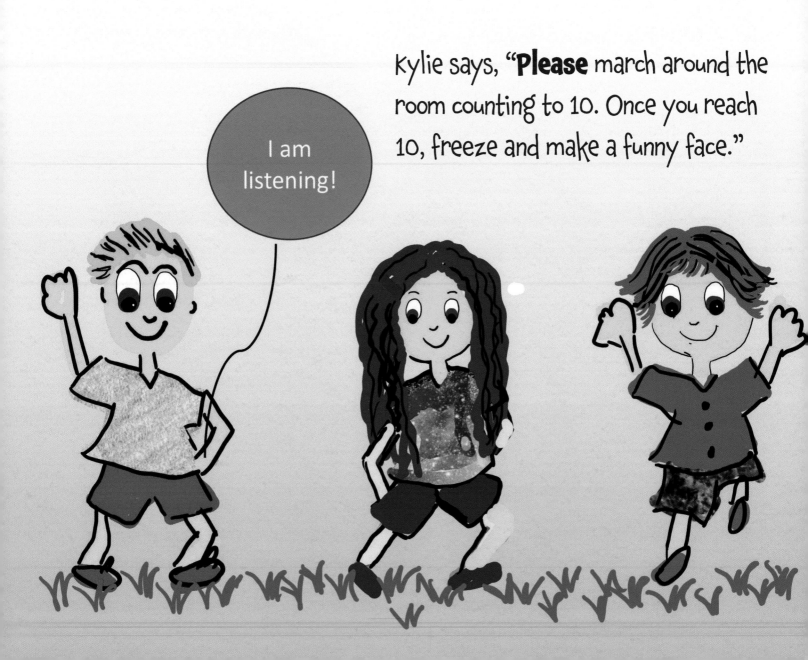

Kylie says, "**Please** shake your hands up high,

Moving is so much fun!

Once you finish, freeze in the shape of a triangle."

then shake them down to the ground. repeat this 5 times.

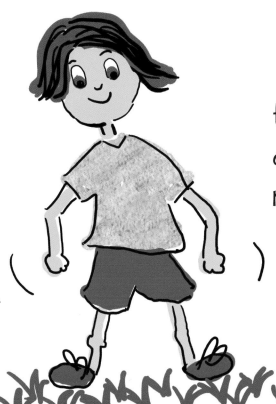
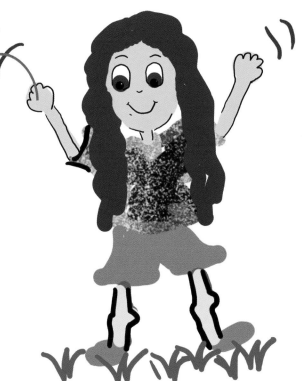

Kylie says, **"Please** pretend you are swimming in the ocean. Uh oh - you see a shark! You'd better swim faster!"

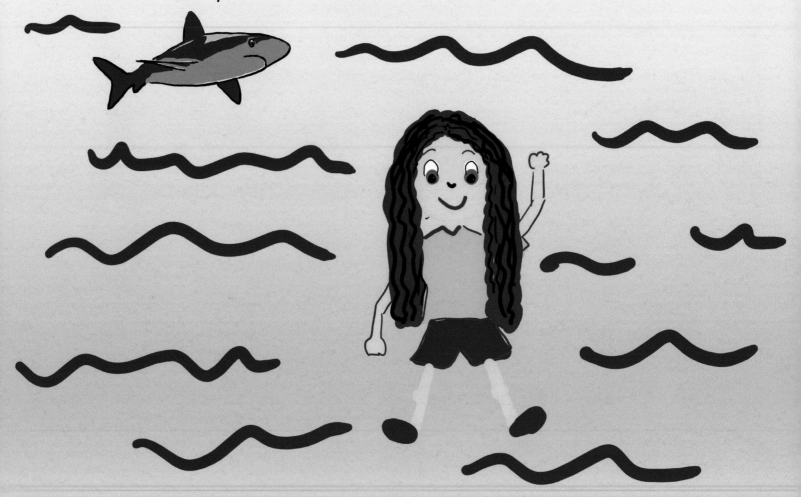

Kylie says, "Do a goofy run.""

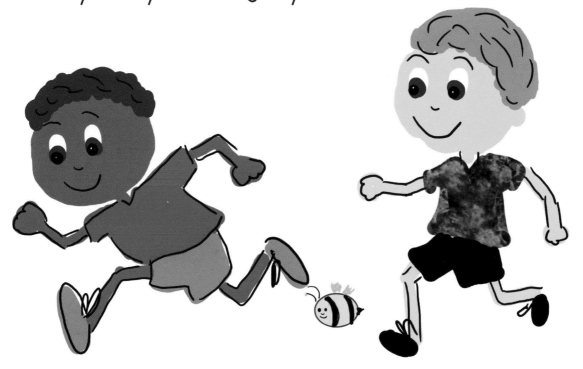

Did Kylie trick you?

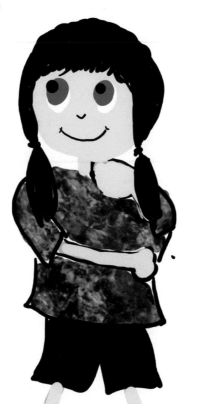

She did not say please.

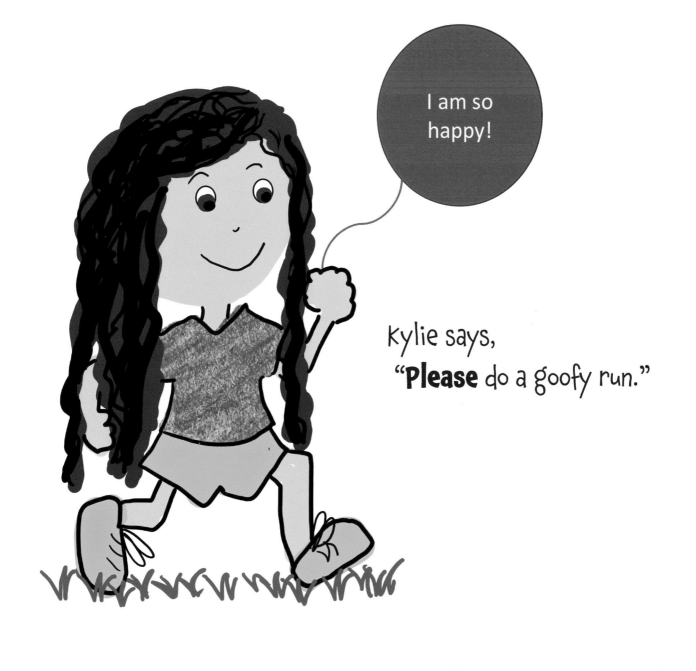

Kylie says,
"**Please** do a goofy run."

Kylie says, "**Please** jump like a frog while making your best frog noise. Freeze on a lily pad after 5 jumps."

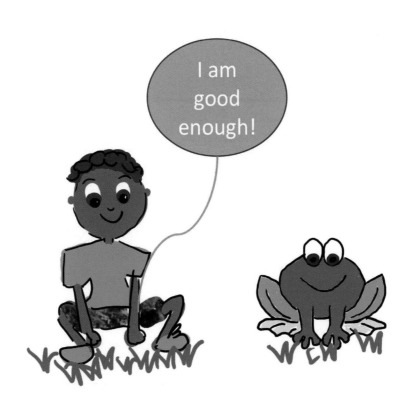

Kylie says, "**Please** glue your feet to the floor and twist your hips."

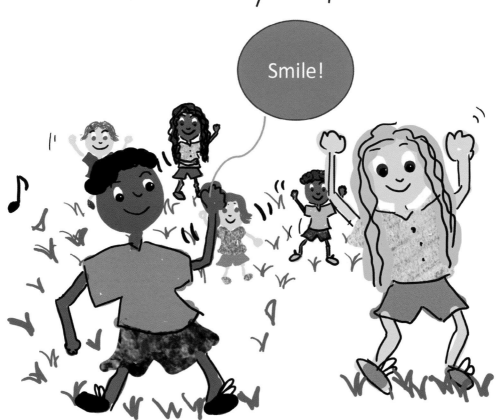

Kylie says,
"**Please** sit criss-cross applesauce."

Peace

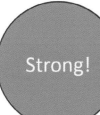 Strong!

Kylie says, "While sitting criss-cross applesauce, **please** try to stand up – without using your hands!"

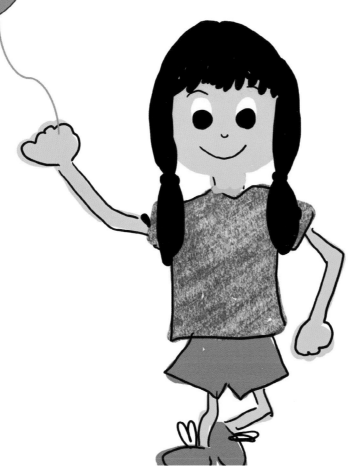

Kylie says, "Jump up and down and wave your arms all around."

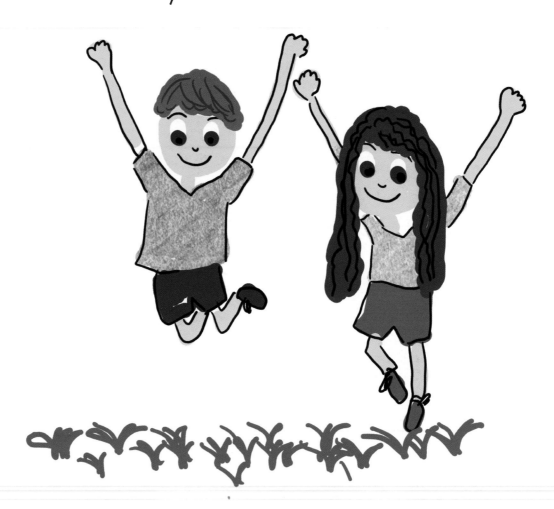

Did Kylie trick you?
Kylie did not say please!

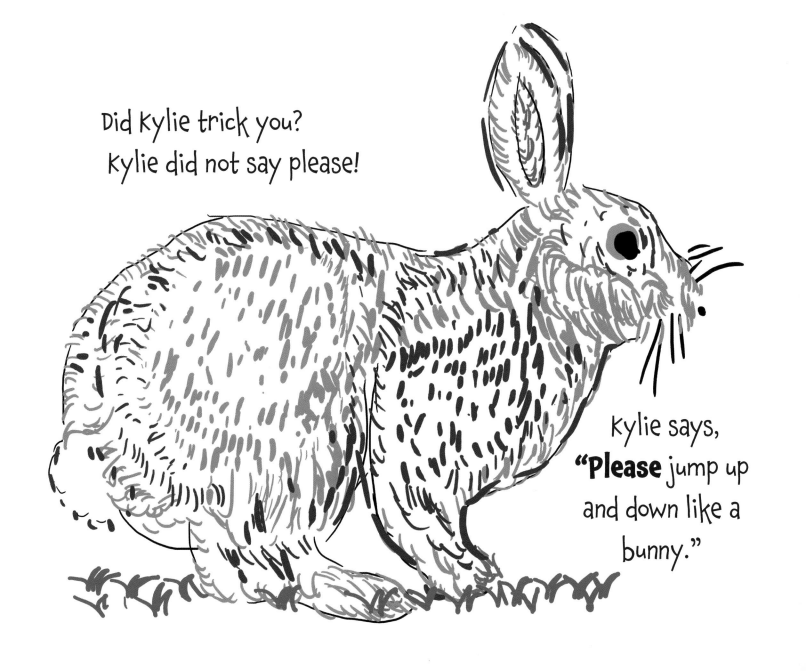

Kylie says,
"Please jump up
and down like a
bunny."

Kylie says, "**Please** do 5 large arm circles forward, and then do 5 large arm circles backwards."

My world is better with you in it!

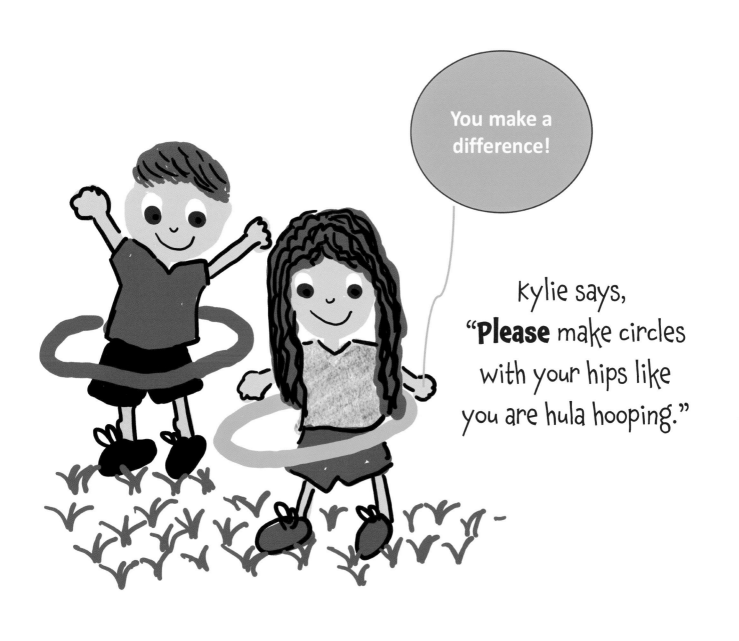

Kylie says, "**Please** make circles with your hips like you are hula hooping."

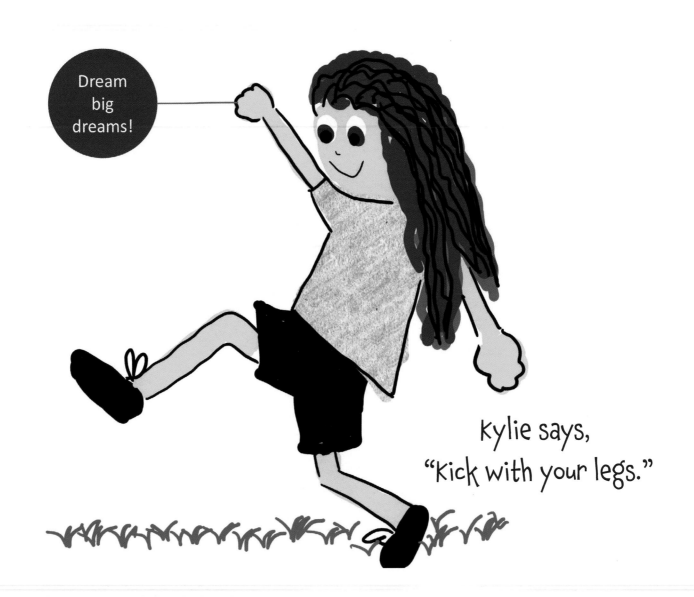

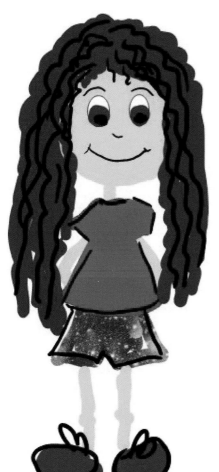

Did Kylie trick you?
She did not say please.

Kylie says, "**Please** kick a pretend football."

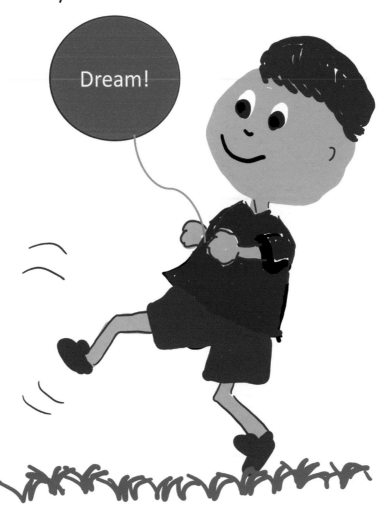

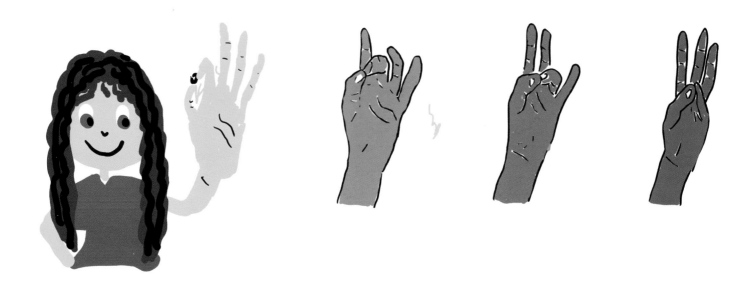

Kylie says, "**Please** touch your thumb to each finger one at a time. Do this with both hands."

Kylie says, "**Please** balance on one foot for 5 seconds, then balance on the other foot for 5 seconds."

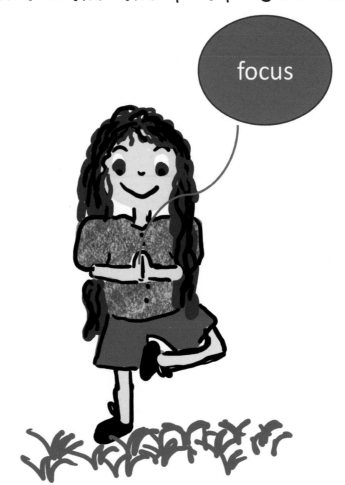

Kylie says, **"Please** skip in a circle."

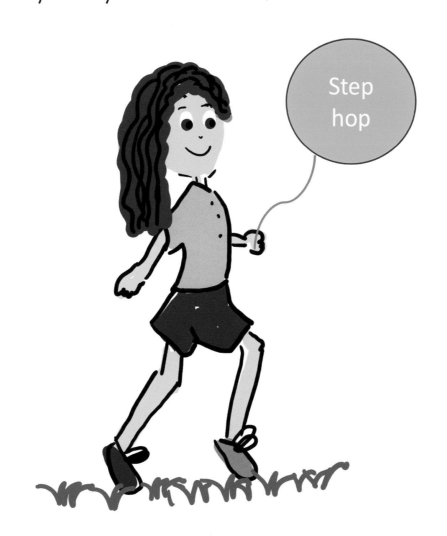

Kylie says, "**Please** pretend you are a puppy dog with a broken leg."

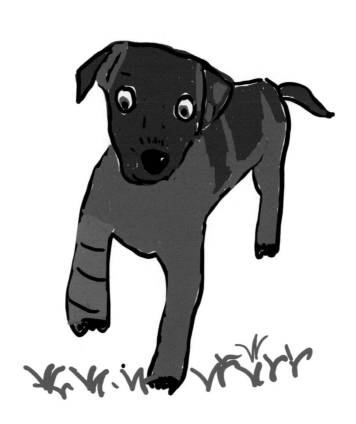

Kylie says, "Stretch up high."

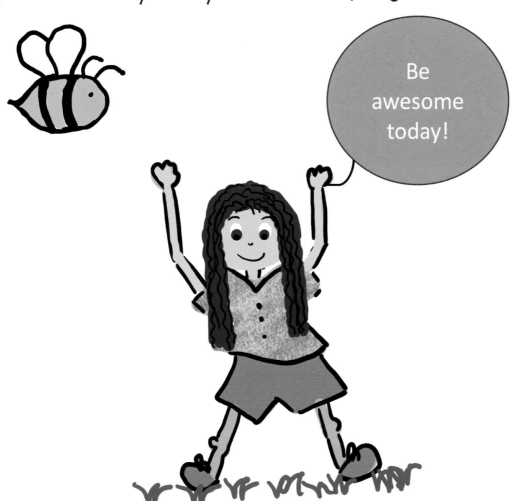

Did Kylie trick you? She has had lots of fun playing today, but now she needs a water break. If you would like to keep playing, choose someone else to be "It." That person can give you actions to do, just like Kylie. Remember though, you only need to do the action if they say the magic word – please!

The End

May you be happy.
May you be healthy.
May you always feel like you belong.